I0842706

This book is dedicated to my daughters Diane and Eliza, and to Christine, their great grandmother who dealt with so much loss but still brought so much joy to the lives of those around her. I wish I had known her better.

Introduction

My journey of motherhood has been an atypical one. At the time of writing this, I have two beautiful, vibrant daughters, 6 and 4. Their pregnancies and deliveries were complication free. Two years after having our second child, we were ready to invite a third into our family, but we experienced 2 devastating miscarriages in succession, followed by over a year of infertility. At the time of writing this book, we were still waiting. Now we're finally pregnant again and can do nothing but hope for the best.

These past 3-4 years have been some of the hardest times of my life. Never have I had such trials of faith, such deep sorrow, and such lack of hope. But also, never have I understood the Atonement and my Savior as deeply as I do now.

I have had some of my deepest struggles with God these last several years, and I was inspired to write this poem after one of those sacred, heart wrenching struggles. The ones when you can't stop asking "why". I pray that my words may resonate with other broken hearts, fathers and mothers alike, who need the reminder that God DOES hear you, whether you've experienced a pregnancy loss or infertility, or both. Sometimes I wish we could flip a switch and end our earthly trials and tribulations, but that would profit us nothing. We must find strength to press forward, even when we have no idea from where that strength will come.

I lie in the dark, quiet hours,
Tears still running down my face.
My arms have been empty far too long.
My womb lacks what it would embrace.

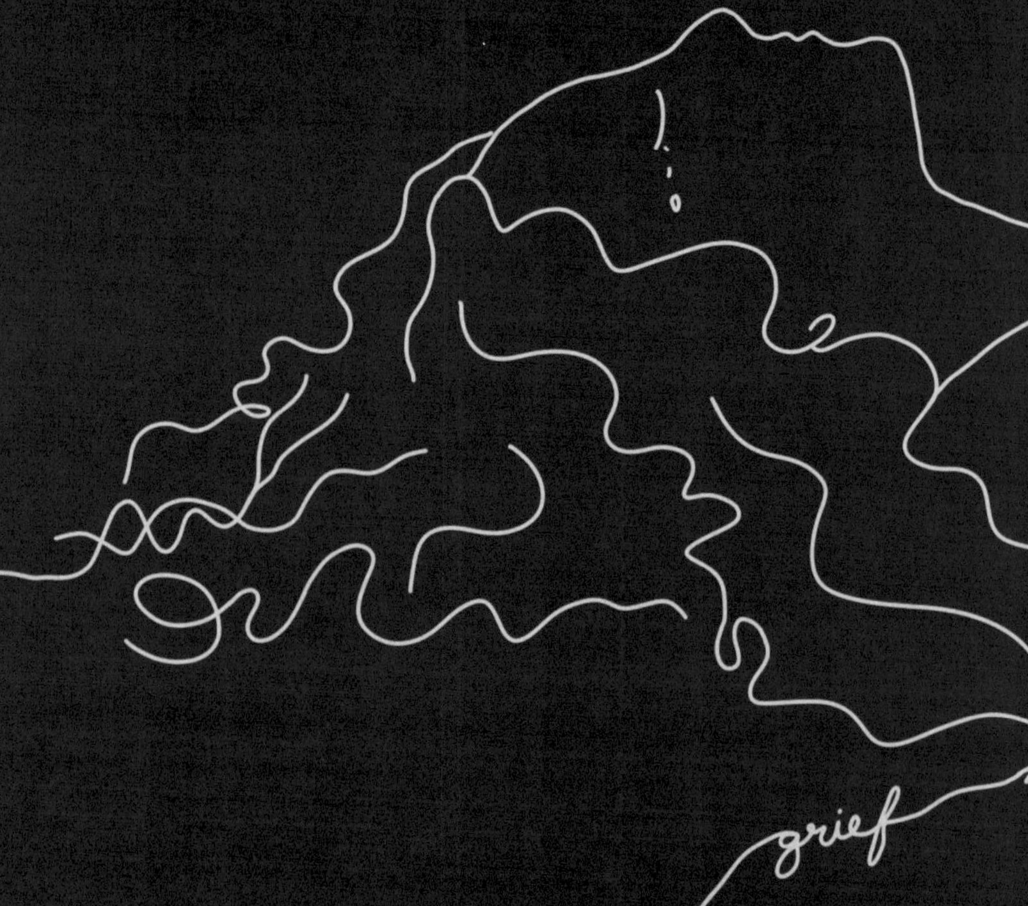

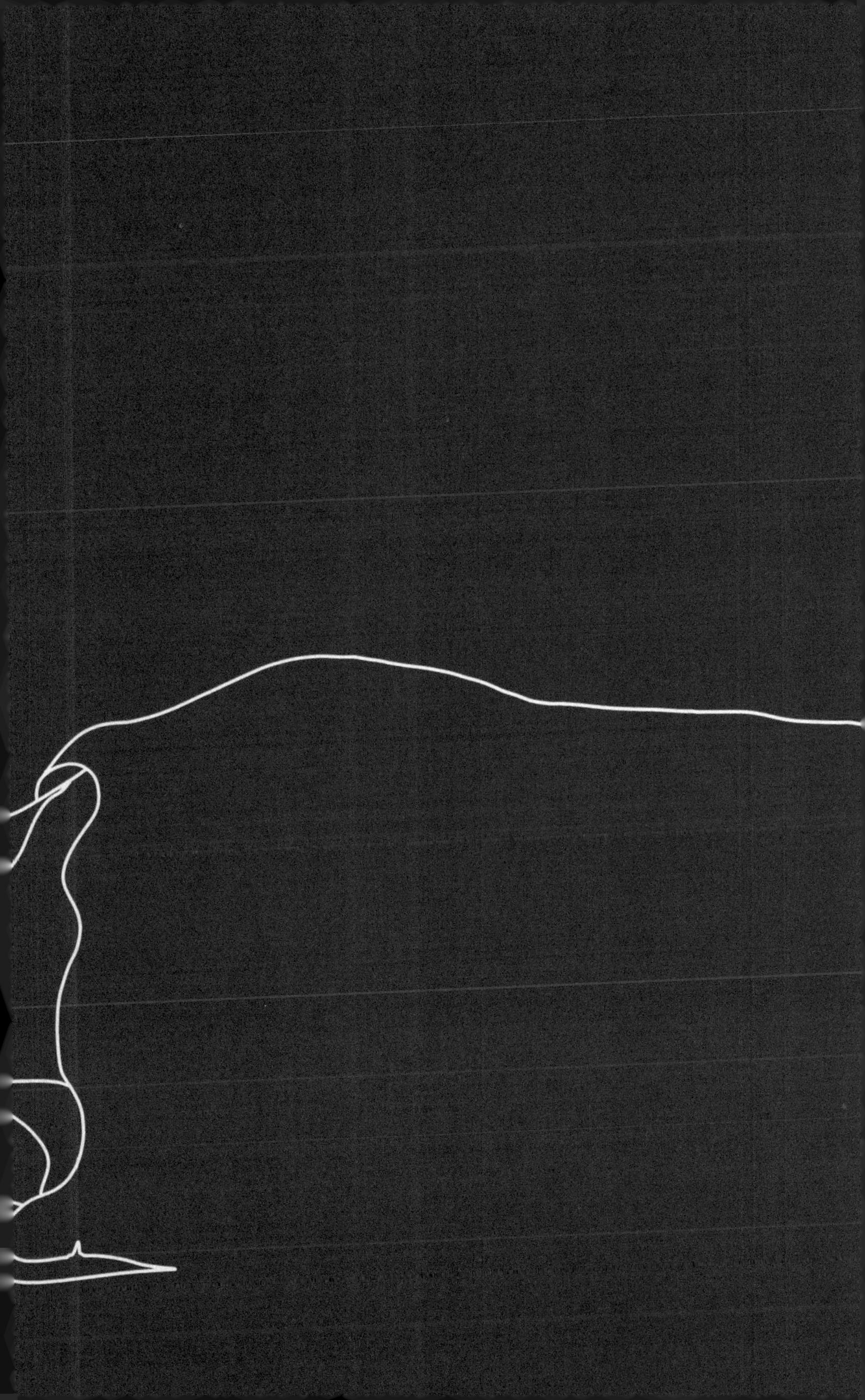

Every month brings on fresh pain.
I question the why, the when, the how.
Will I *ever* carry another child?

Grief and loss consume me now.

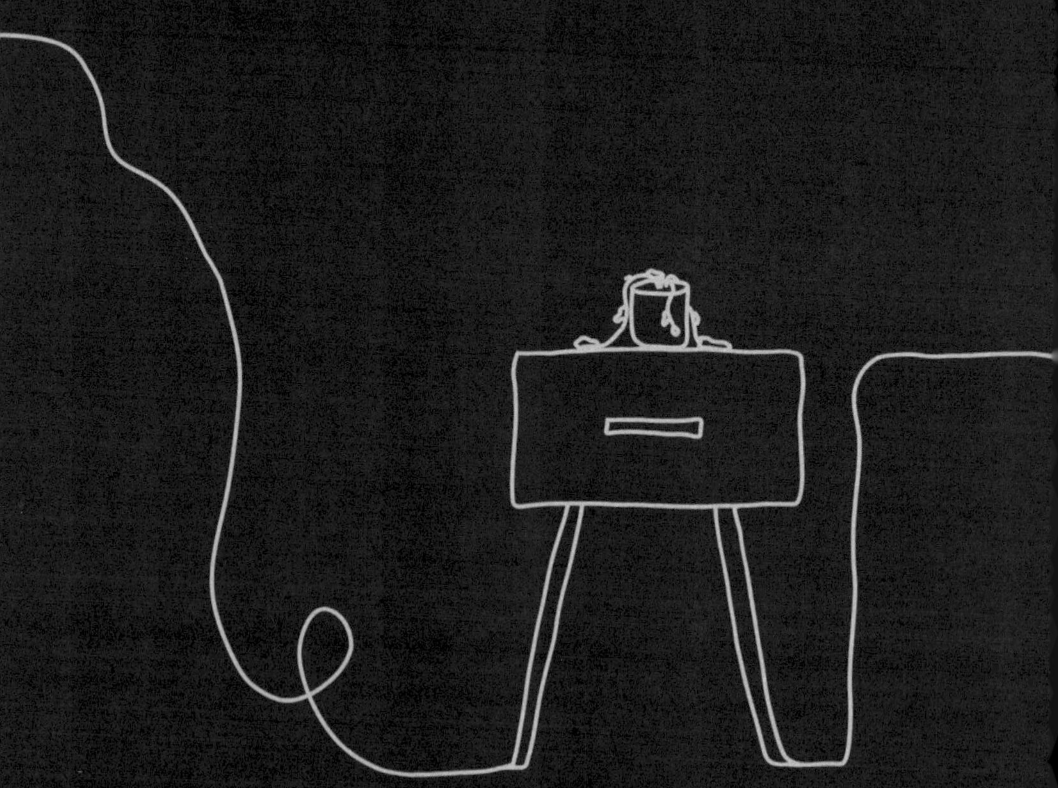

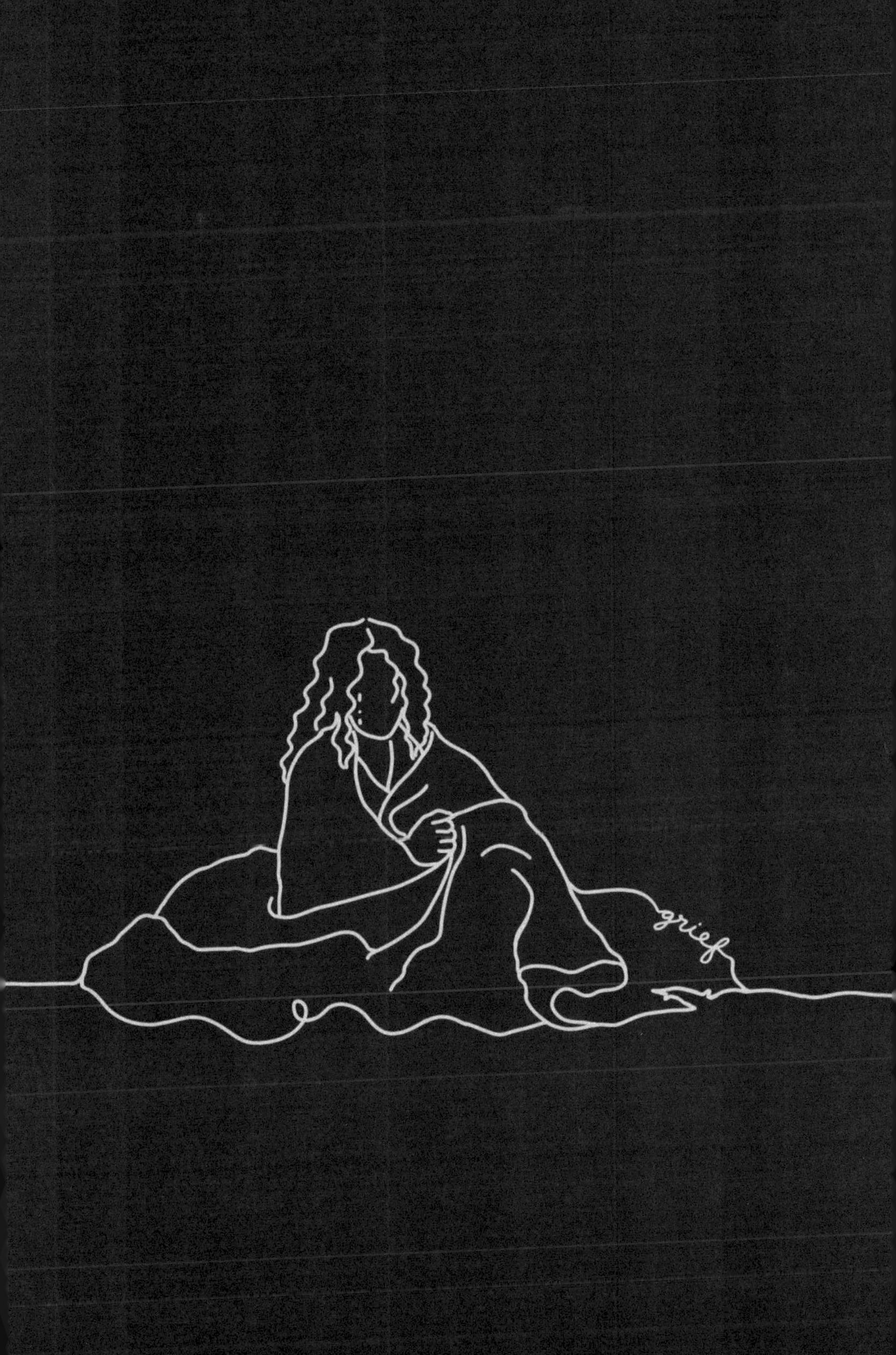
grief

I sit up and face myself,
And reach my heart to heav'n in prayer:

Father, Savior, Heavenly Mother,

Are you *listening?*

Do you *care?*

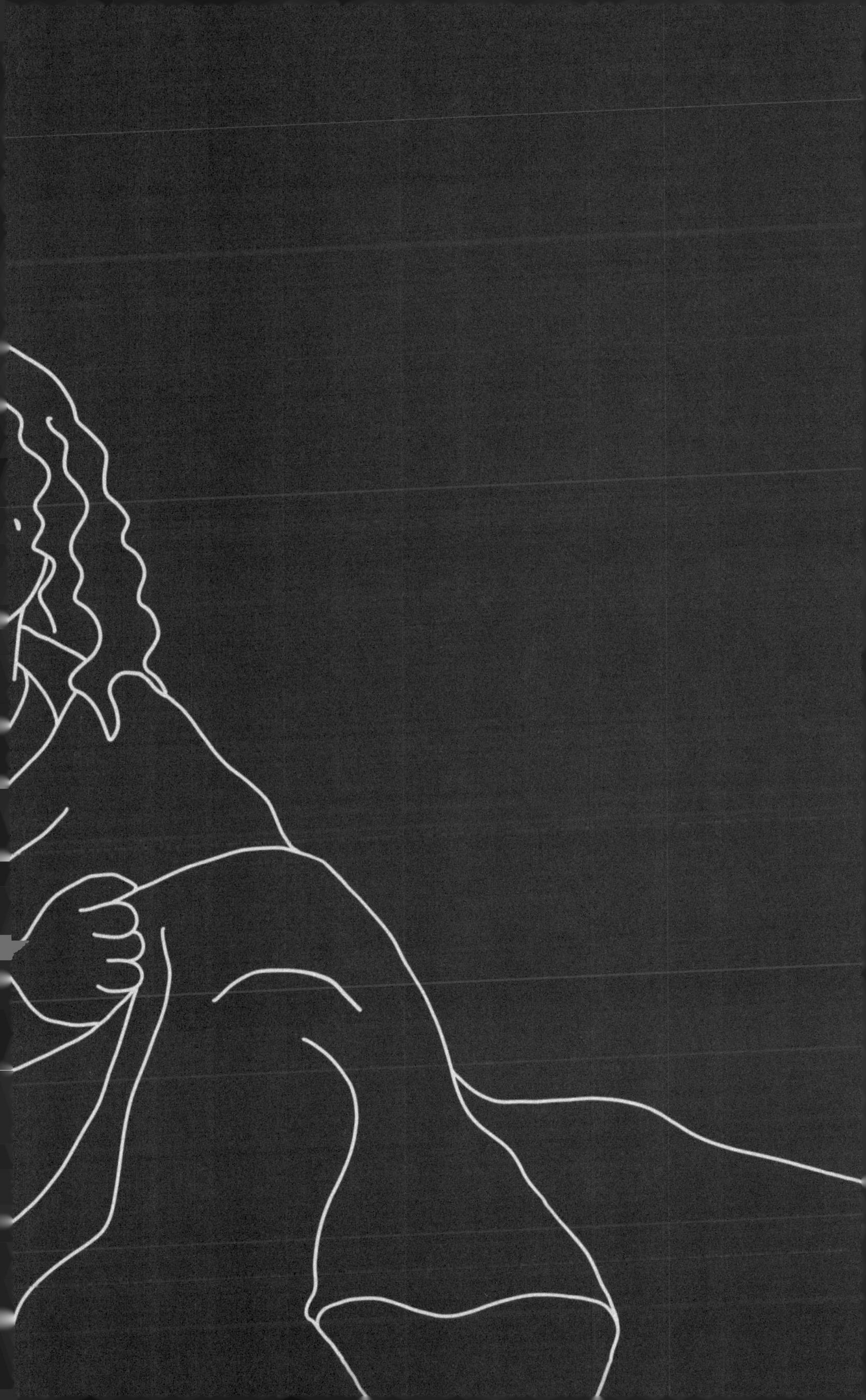

Why have you not answered me?
Is this not a righteous, true desire?
Am I doomed to close my heart?
Is all hope gone? My soul is tired...

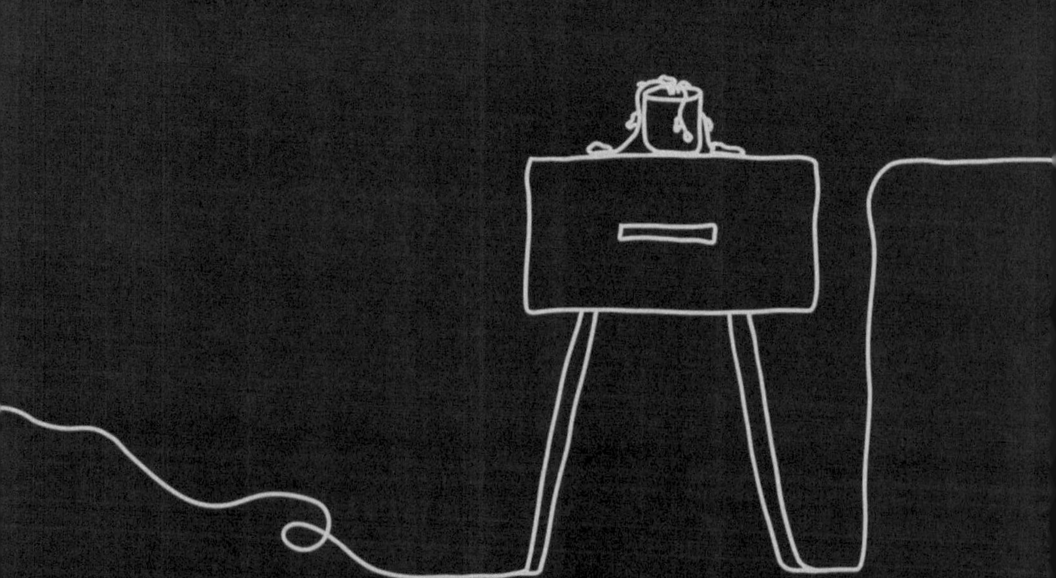

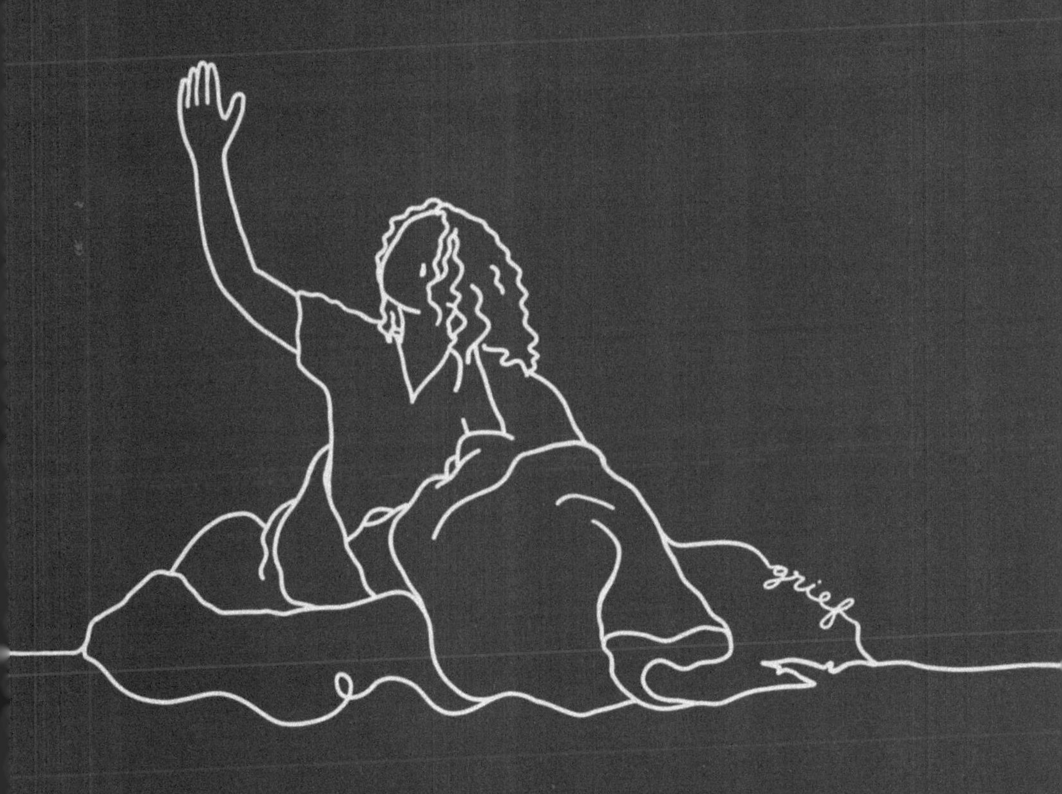
grief

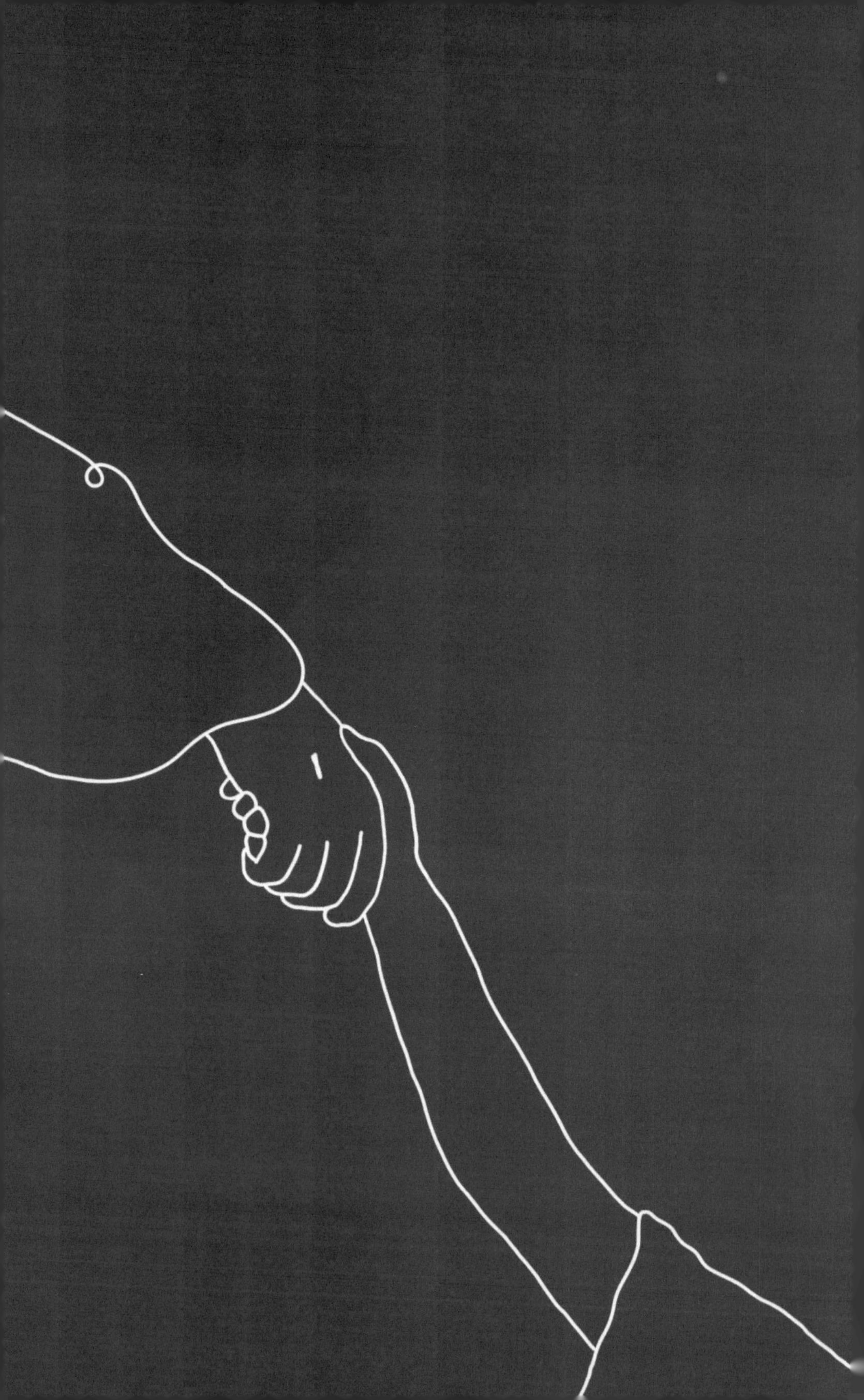

I am here.

My Little One, *Jesus whispers,*
Lay down your grief, I've felt it too.
I know your pain. I've also been

In a place as *dark* and low as *you.*

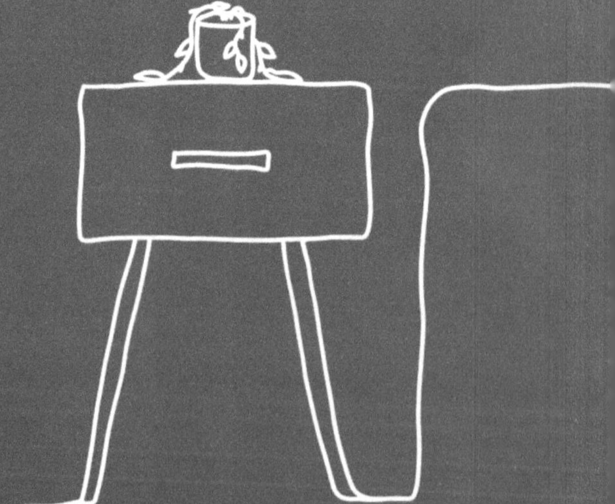

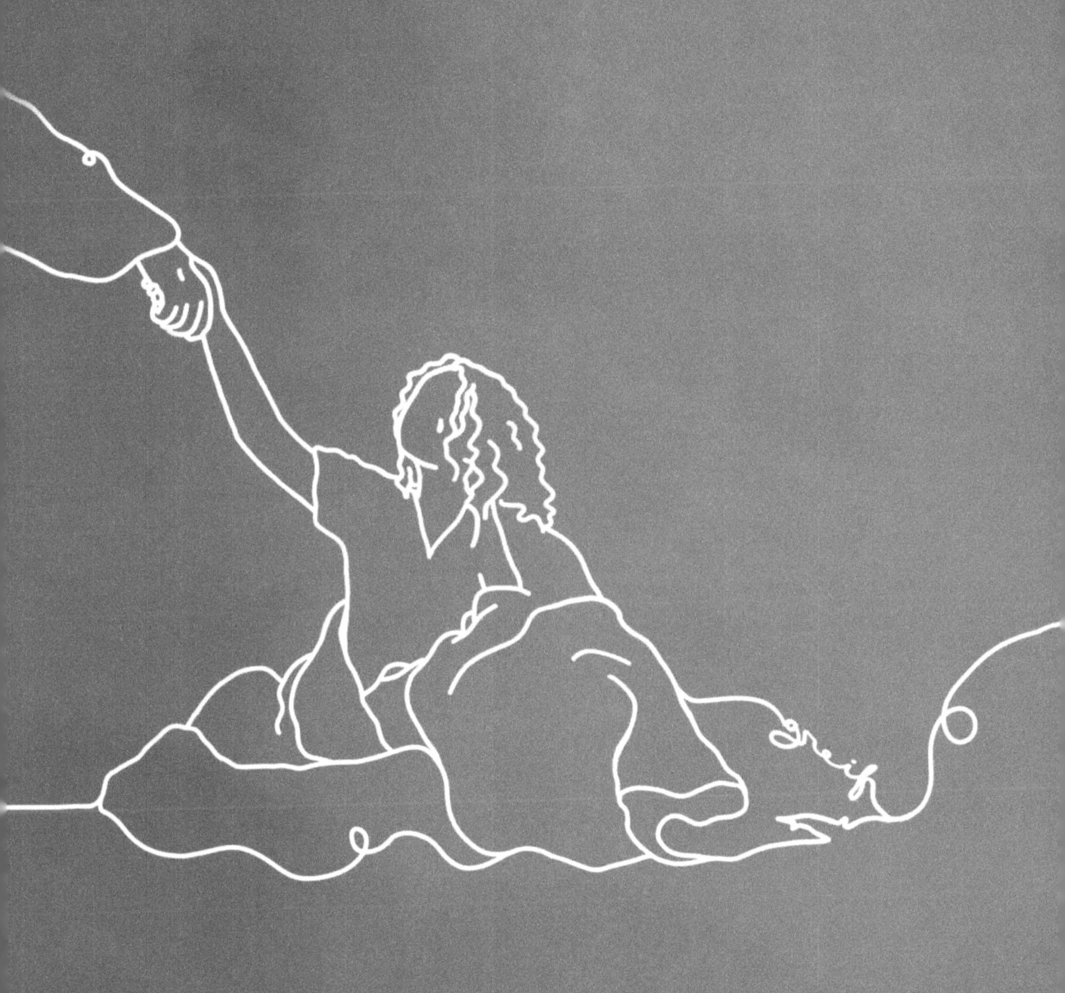

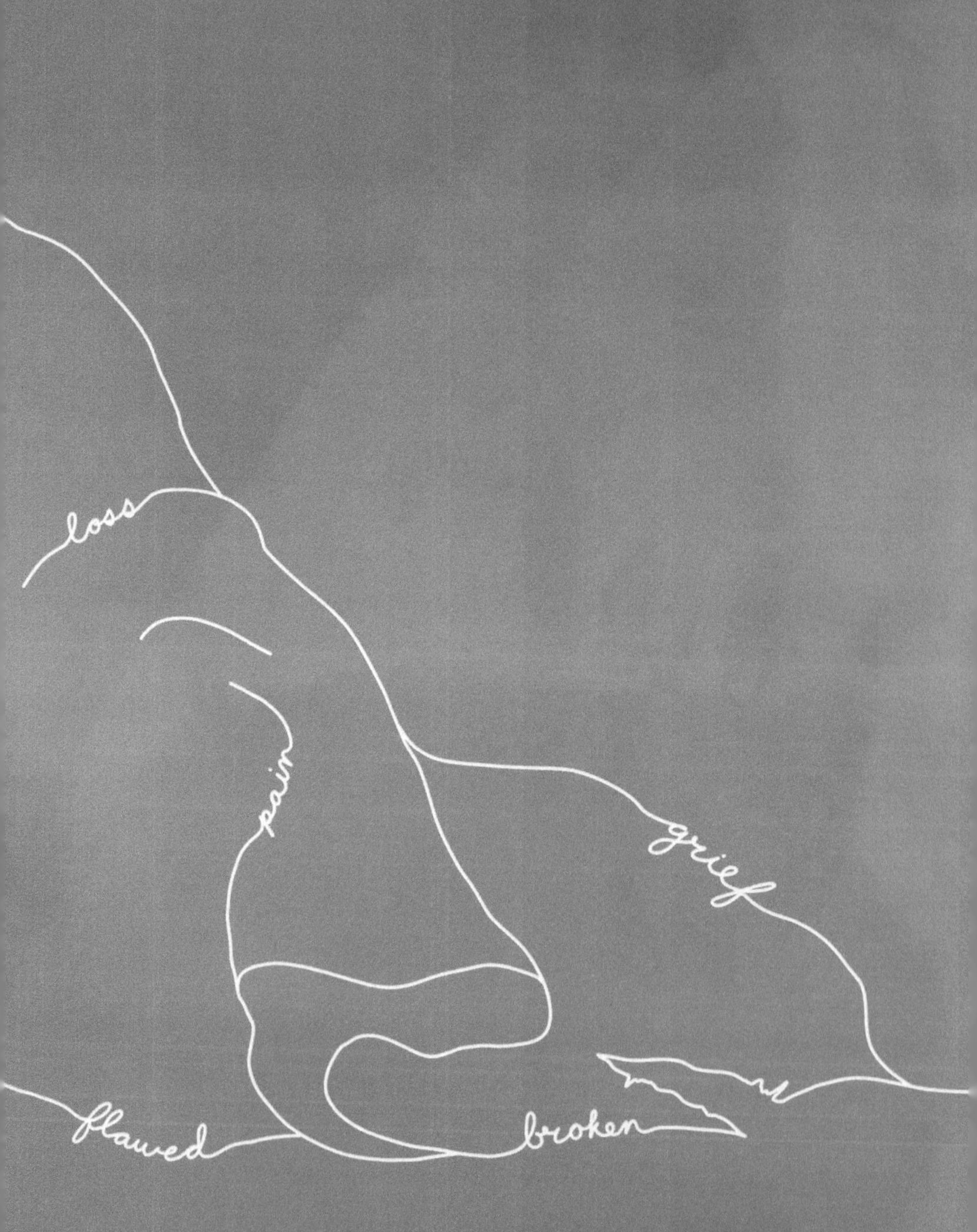
loss
pain
grief
flawed
broken

Look at yourself, your worth, your heart.
You are heard and understood,

But the world is fallen and flawed, my dear,
And nature rolls forth as it would.

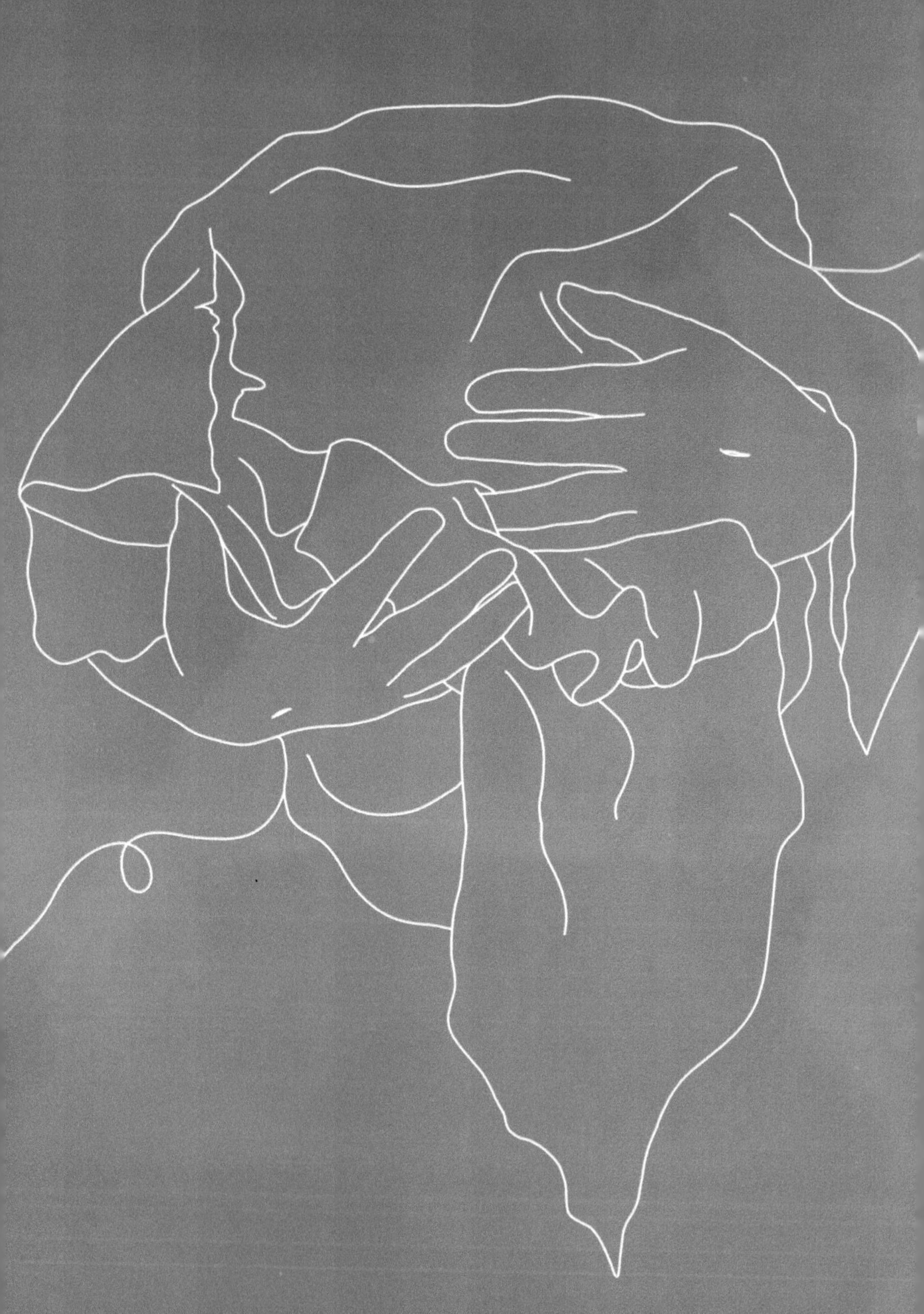

I cannot take away your trials,
  But I can help you *carry* them.

  If you will just lay down your *grief,*
I'll pick it up and hold it, too.

Then you can stand up *free* of pain
You'll still remember, but will not cry.
Through my grace, your heart can heal.

It's possible, if you will *try.*

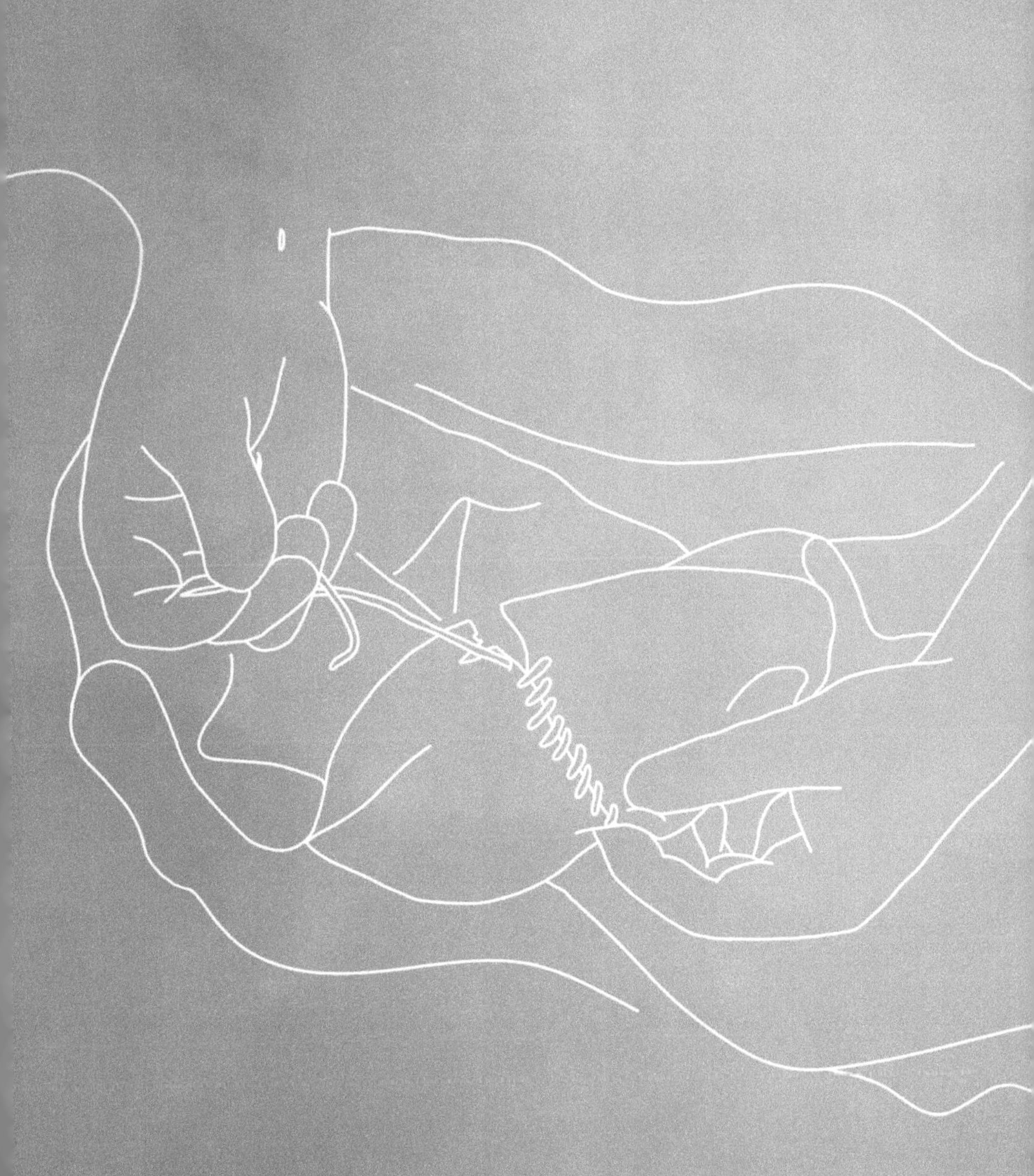

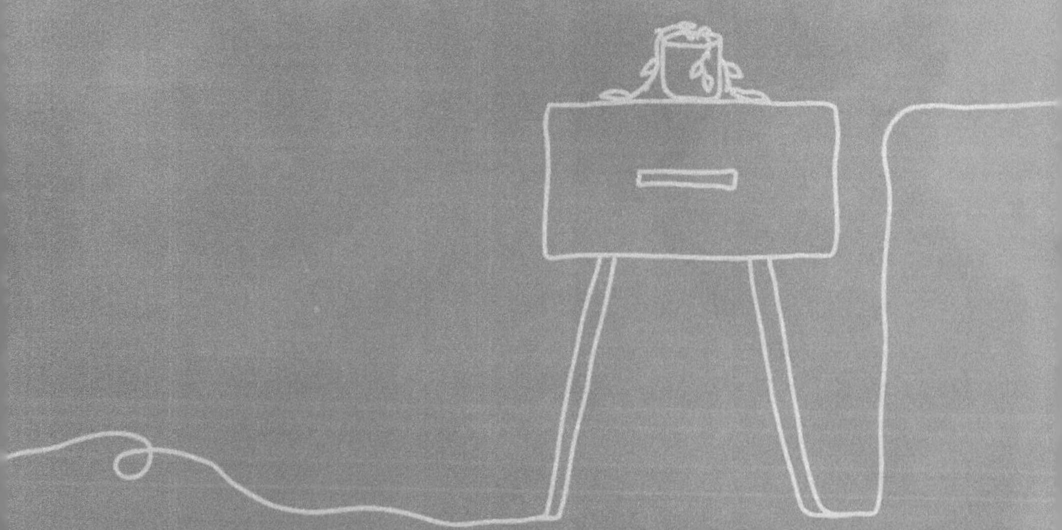

No, I say.

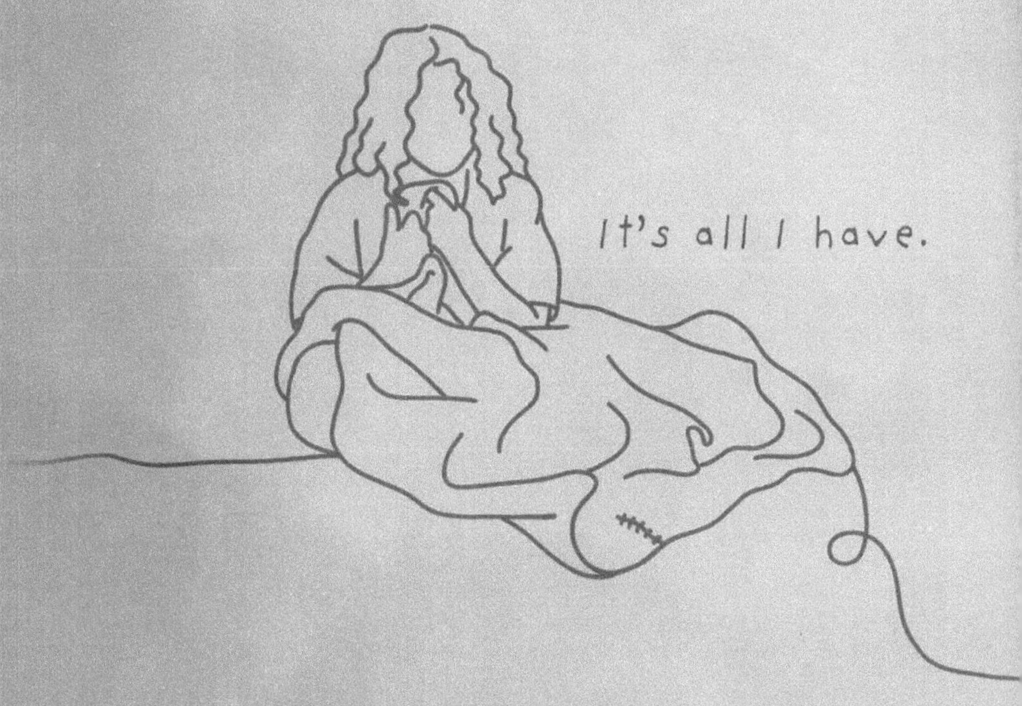
It's all I have.

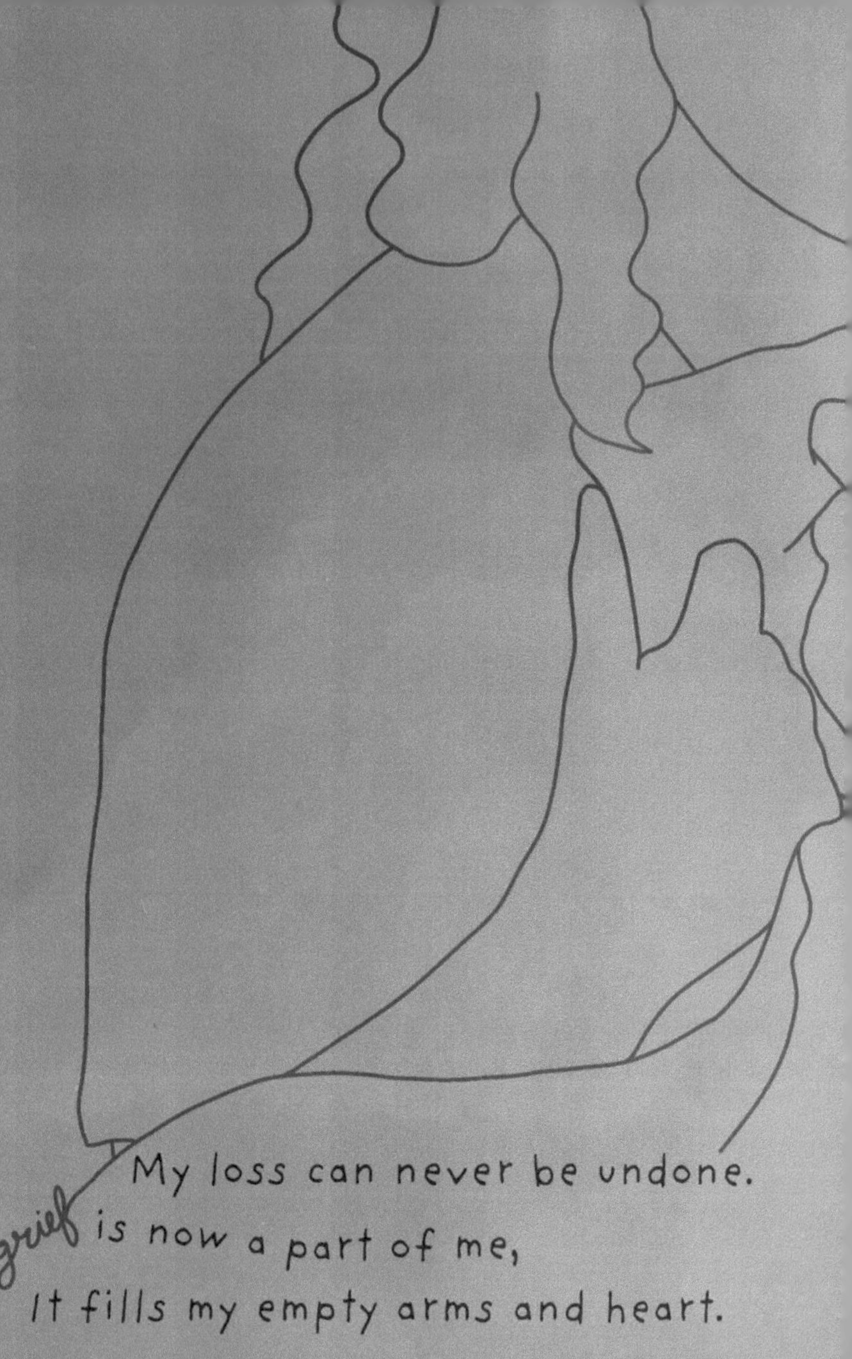

My loss can never be undone.
The grief is now a part of me,
It fills my empty arms and heart.

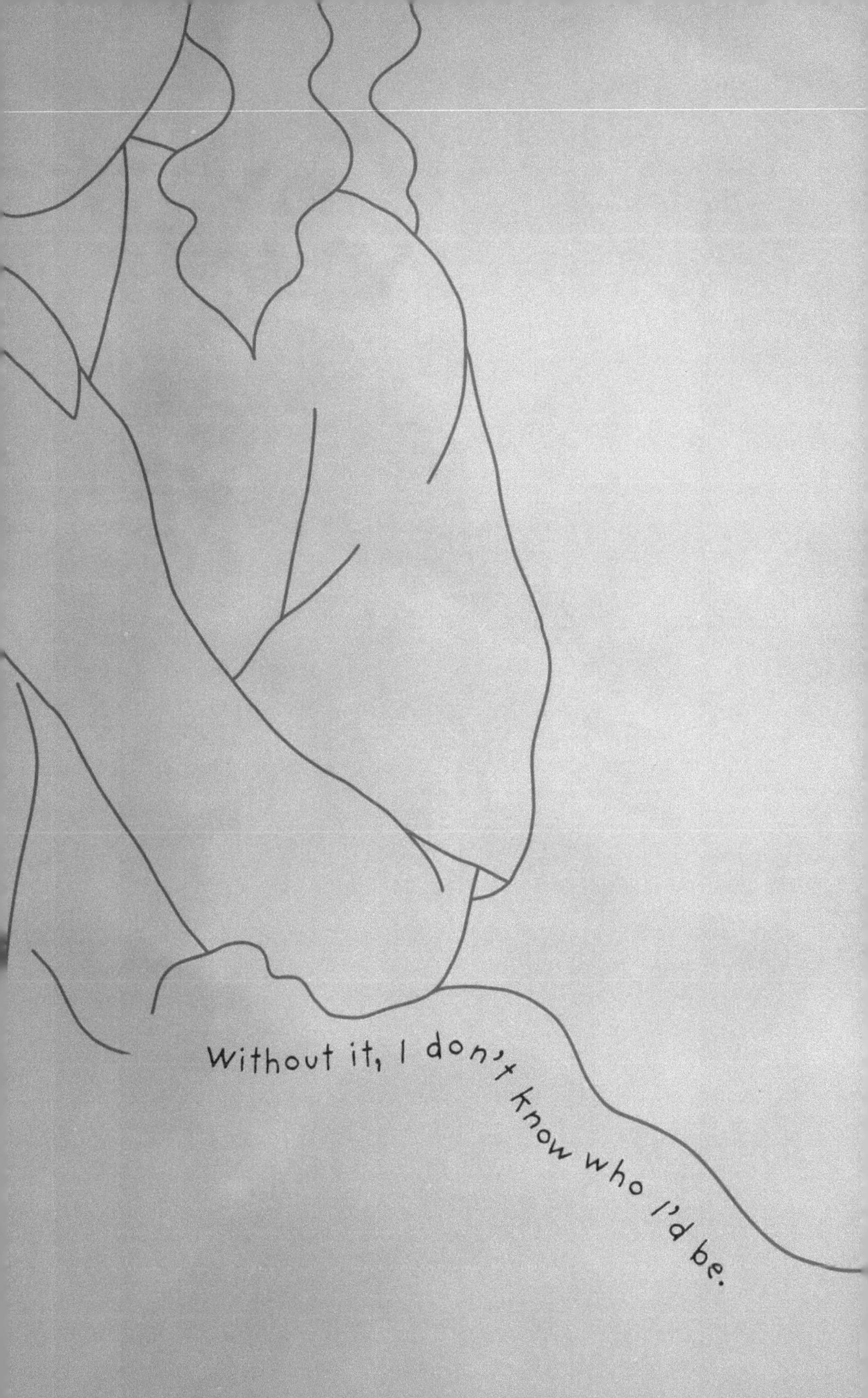

Without it, I don't know who I'd be.

Lay down your grief and trust in me.
Again, his words come soft and low,

Carrying darkness will dim the light
You need for your own soul to *grow*.

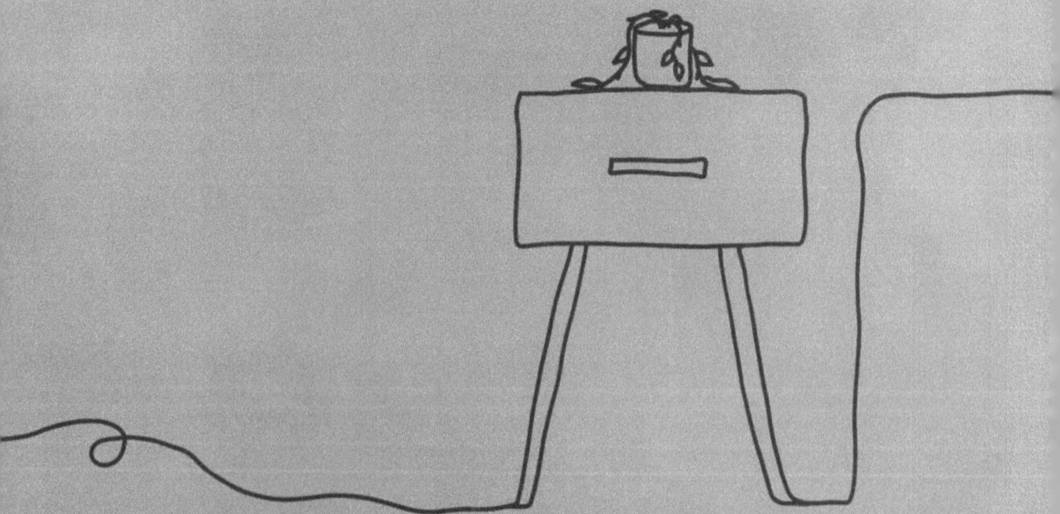

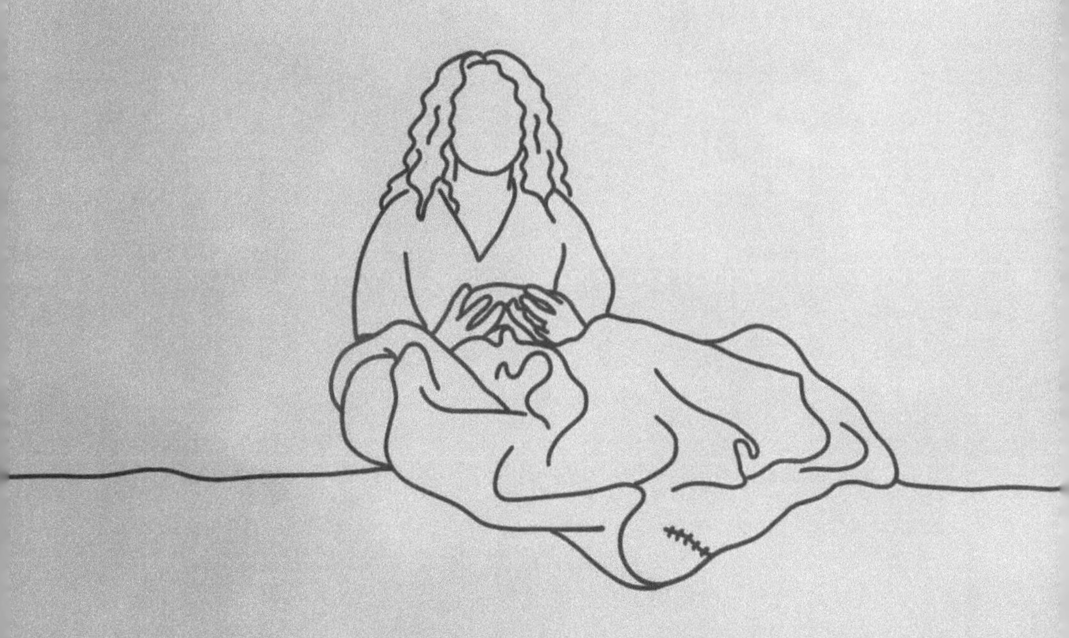

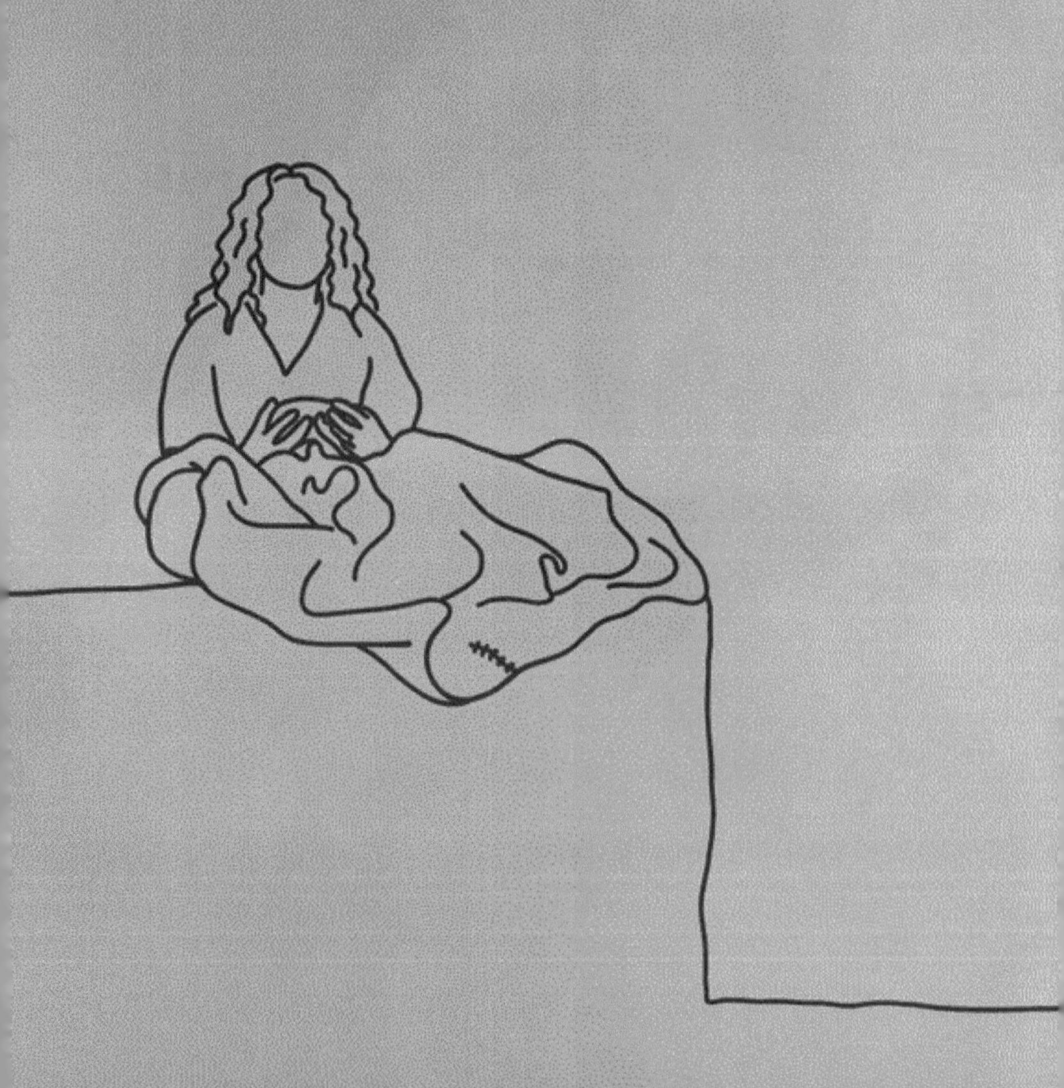

Hold on to what you cherish most:
Your *family,*
your *service,*
your *joy,*
Then hold on tighter to your *faith,*
For sorrow can your faith destroy.

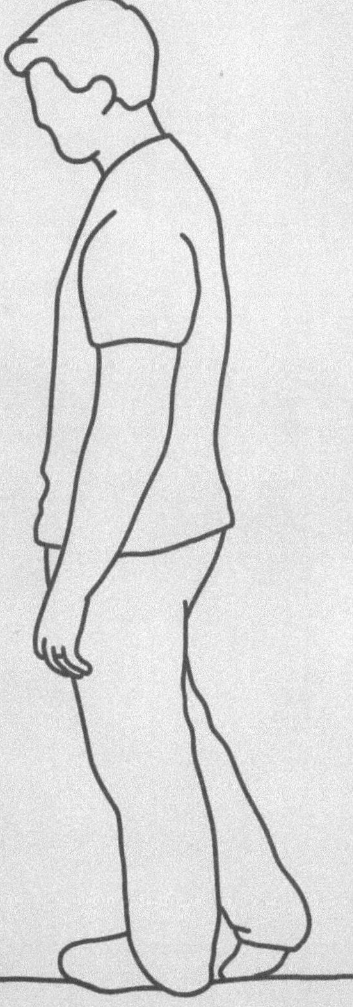

Though you can't see what the future holds,
Be of good courage, for *you are seen.*

You are doing well, my dear.
Get up and *just* keep moving.

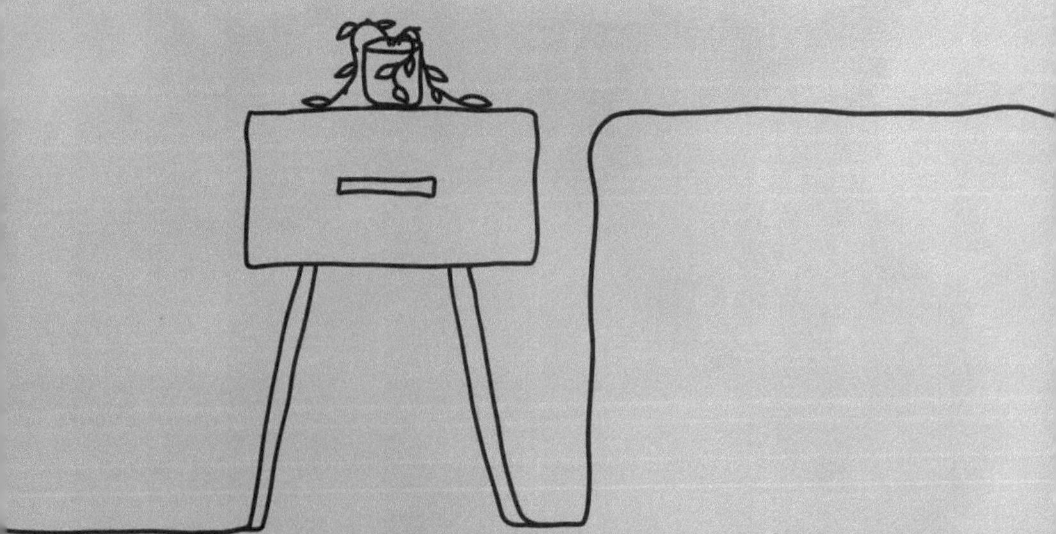

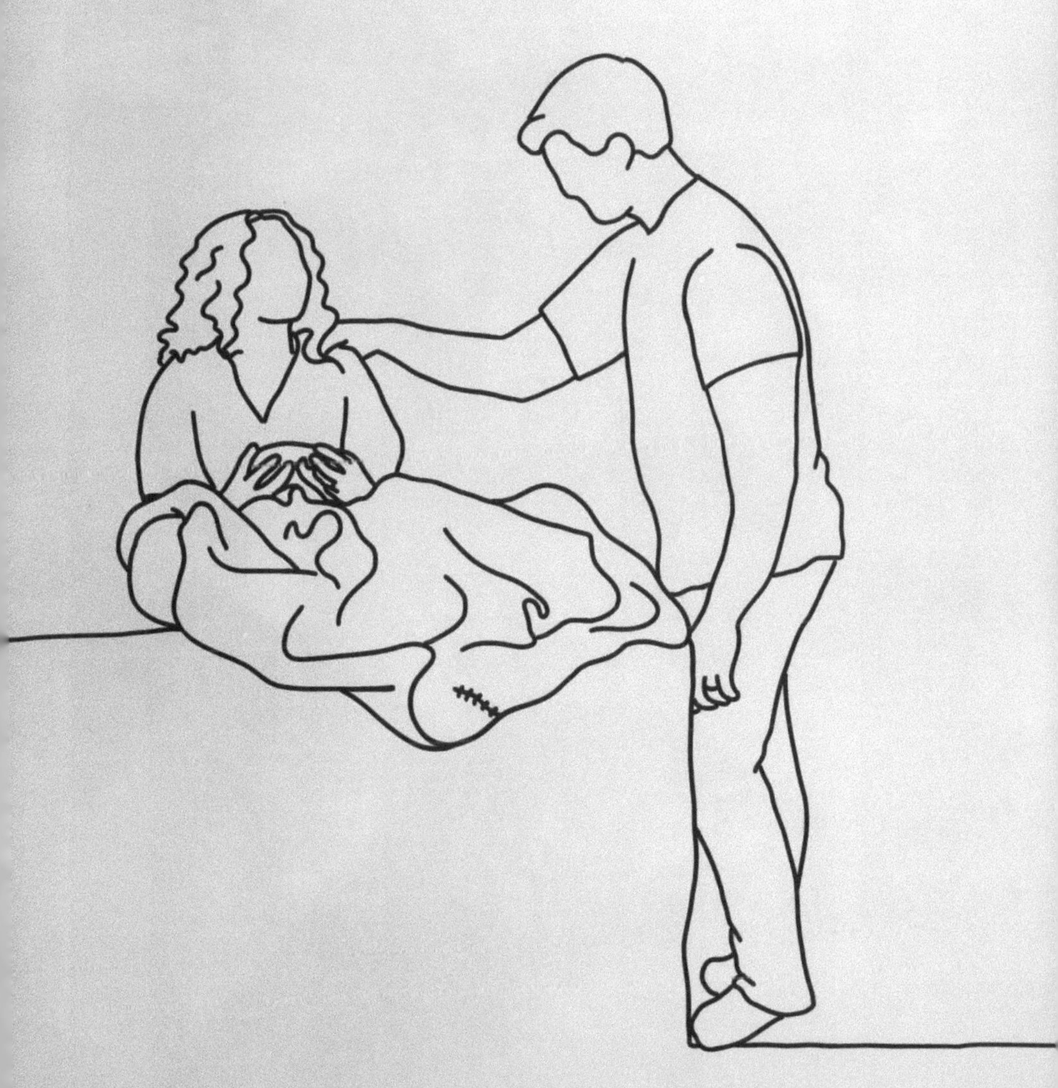

And when the weight is heavy again,

Look *up*,

look *in*,

look *out*.

There is still *value* in what you have,
Which you'll see if you look about.

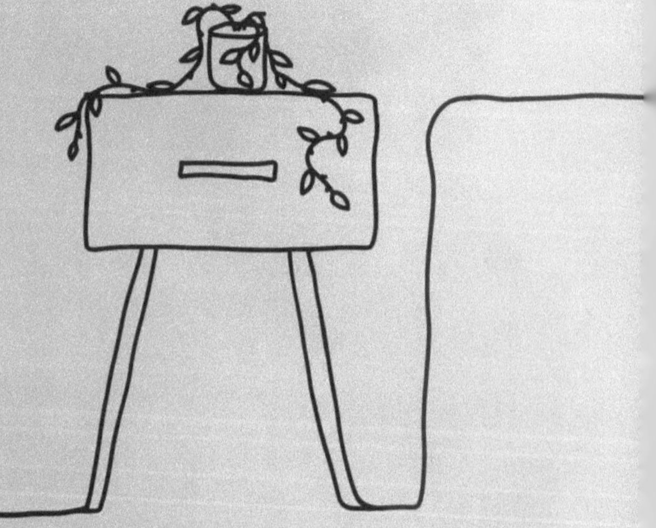

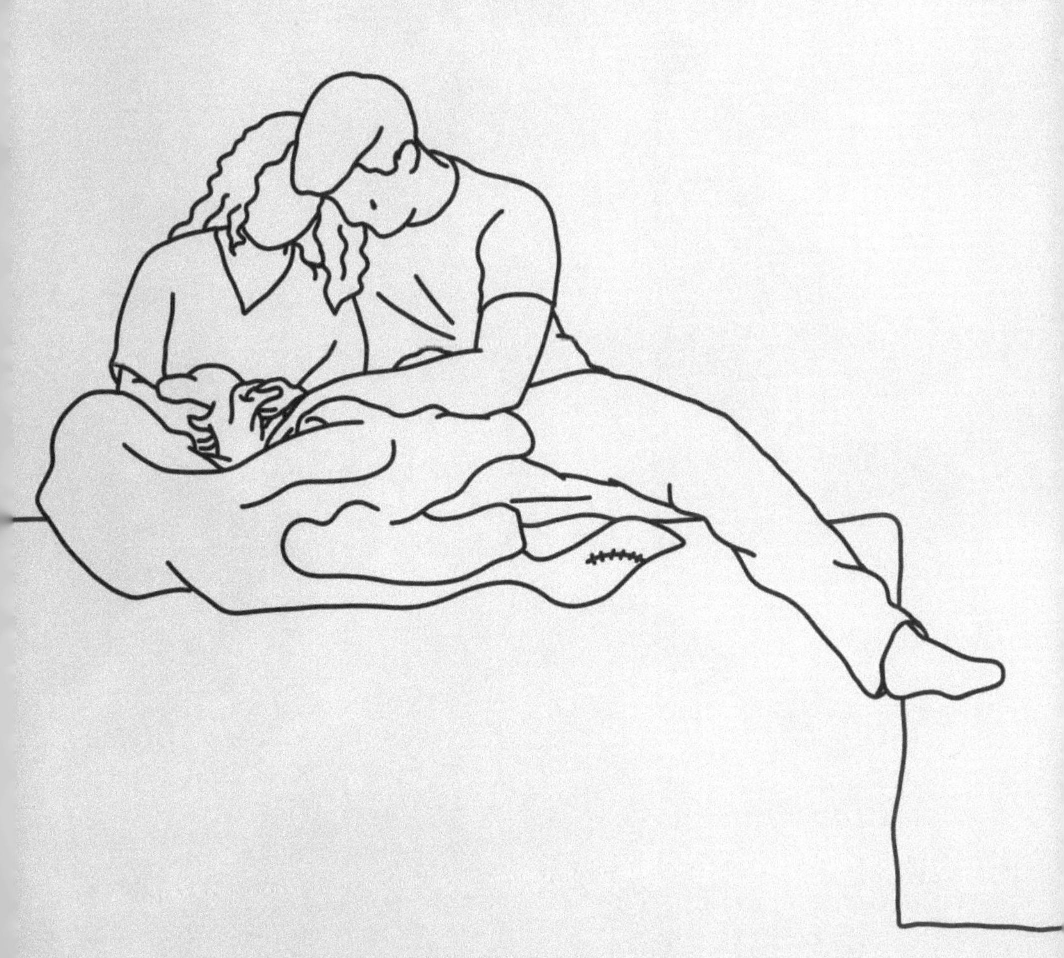

And at first,

It will take *work*,

But you'll learn to trust in me *again*;

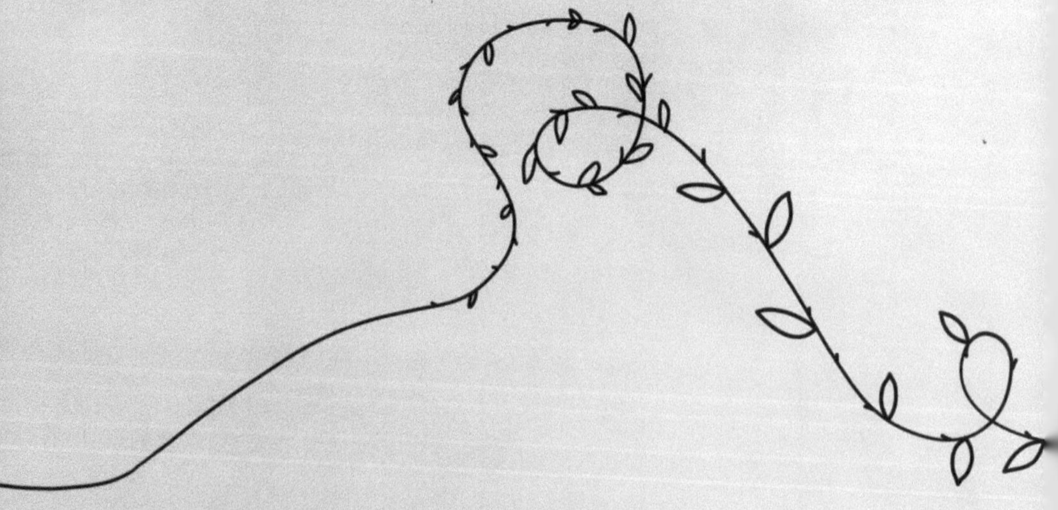

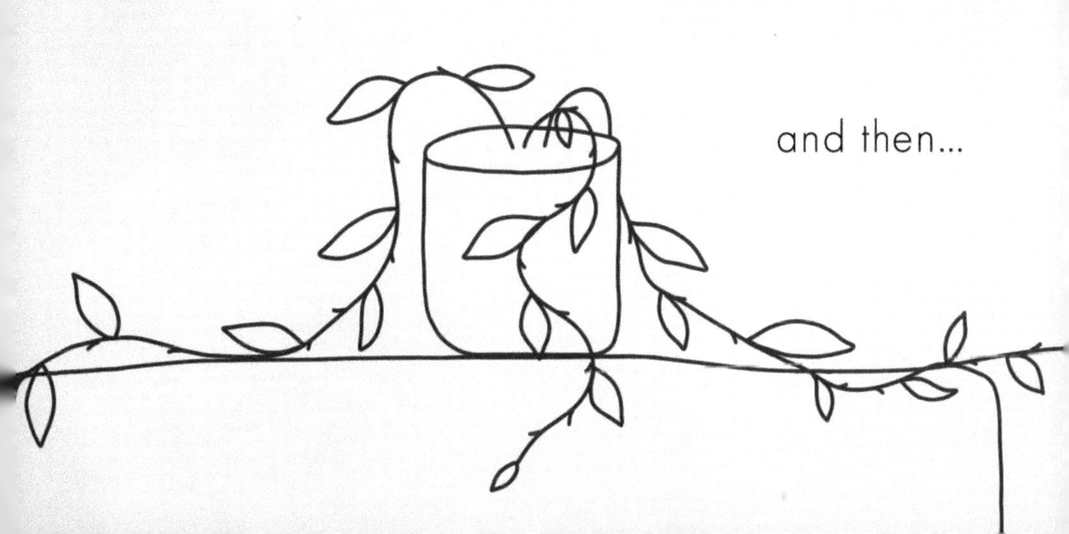

and then...

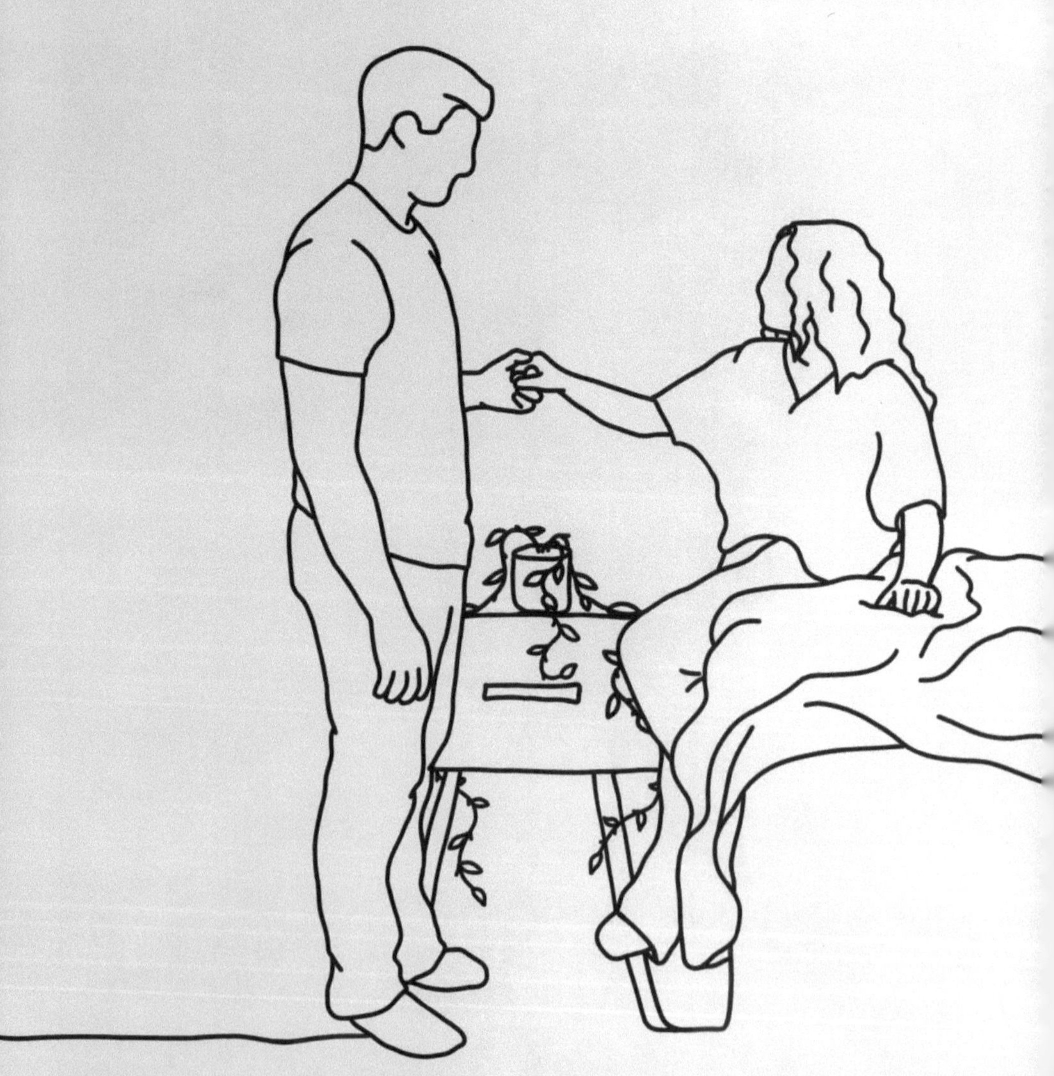

If the blessing you so dearly seek,
Does not come as you hoped it would,

Keep *working,*
keep *trying,*
keep *serving* on.

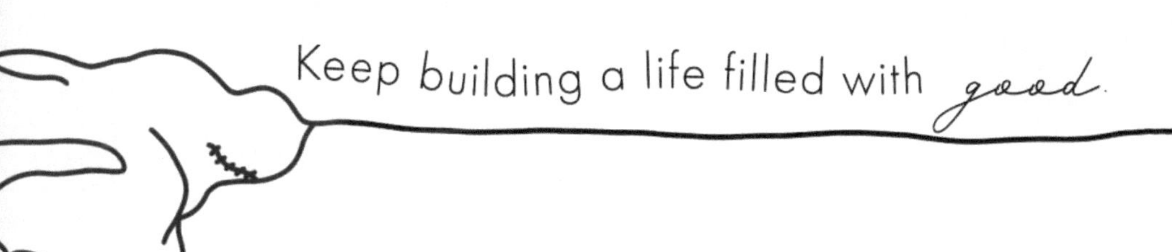

Keep building a life filled with *good.*

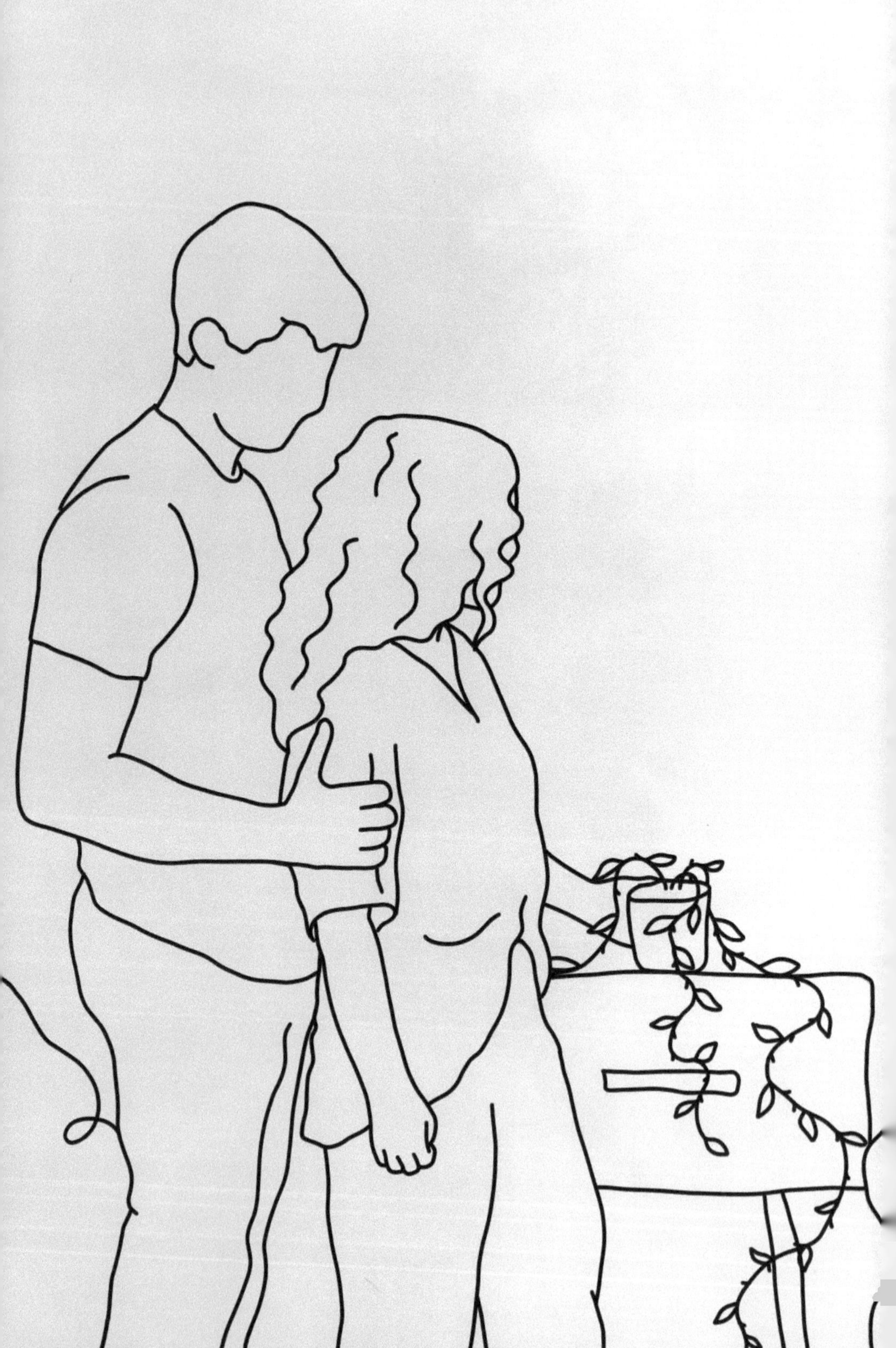

Eternity is a long, long time.

And the babes you've lost along your way
Will *always* be a part of you,

No matter what others say.

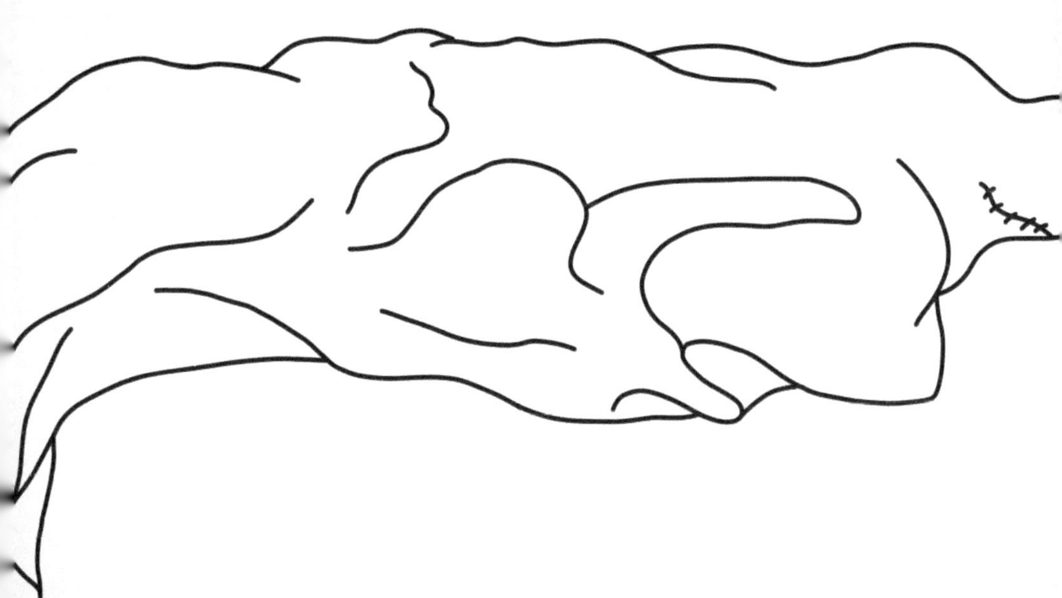

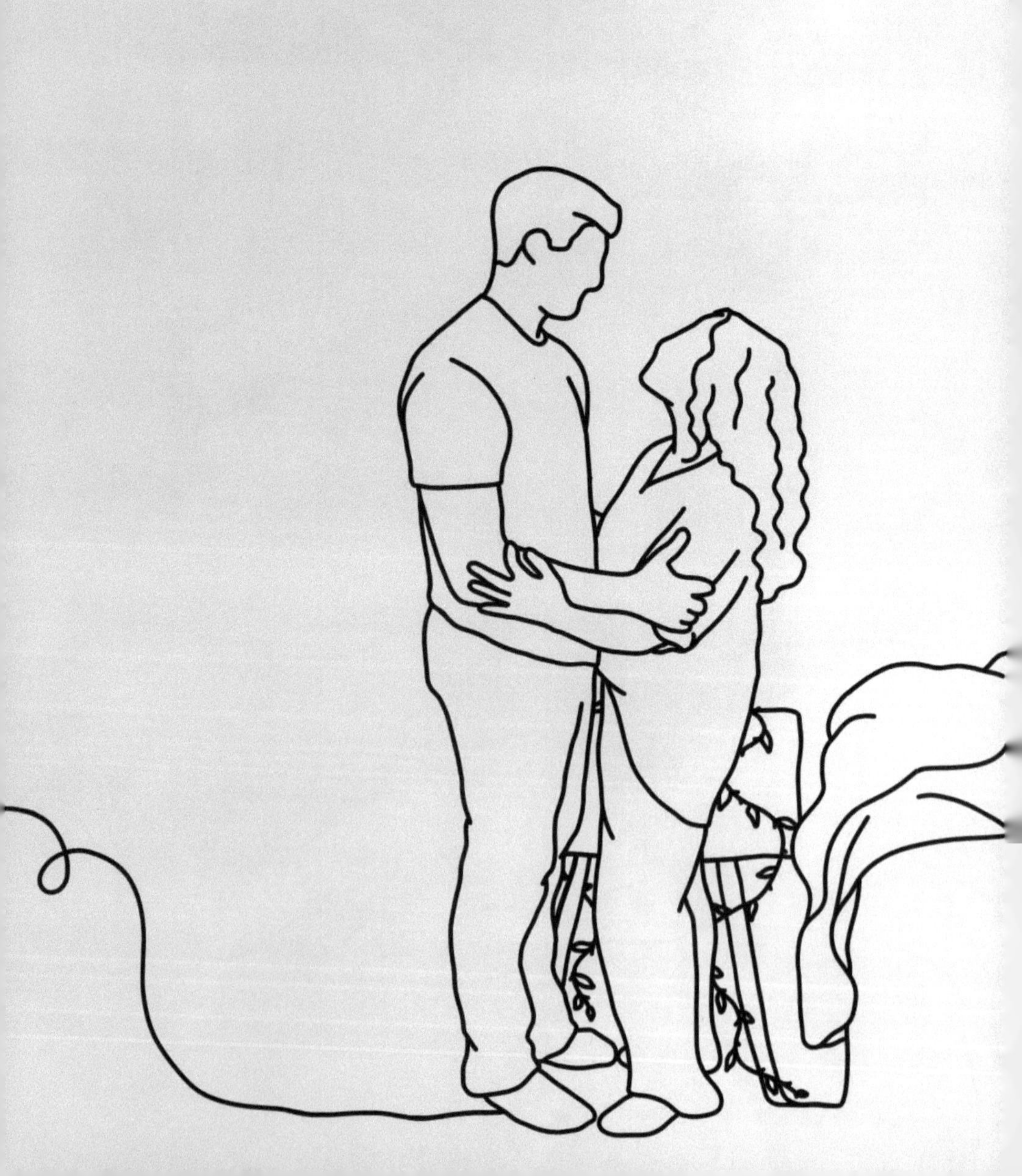

And *I* will hold you through it all,
And you'll become who you should be.
A loving mother of precious souls,

Bound *together* for eternity.

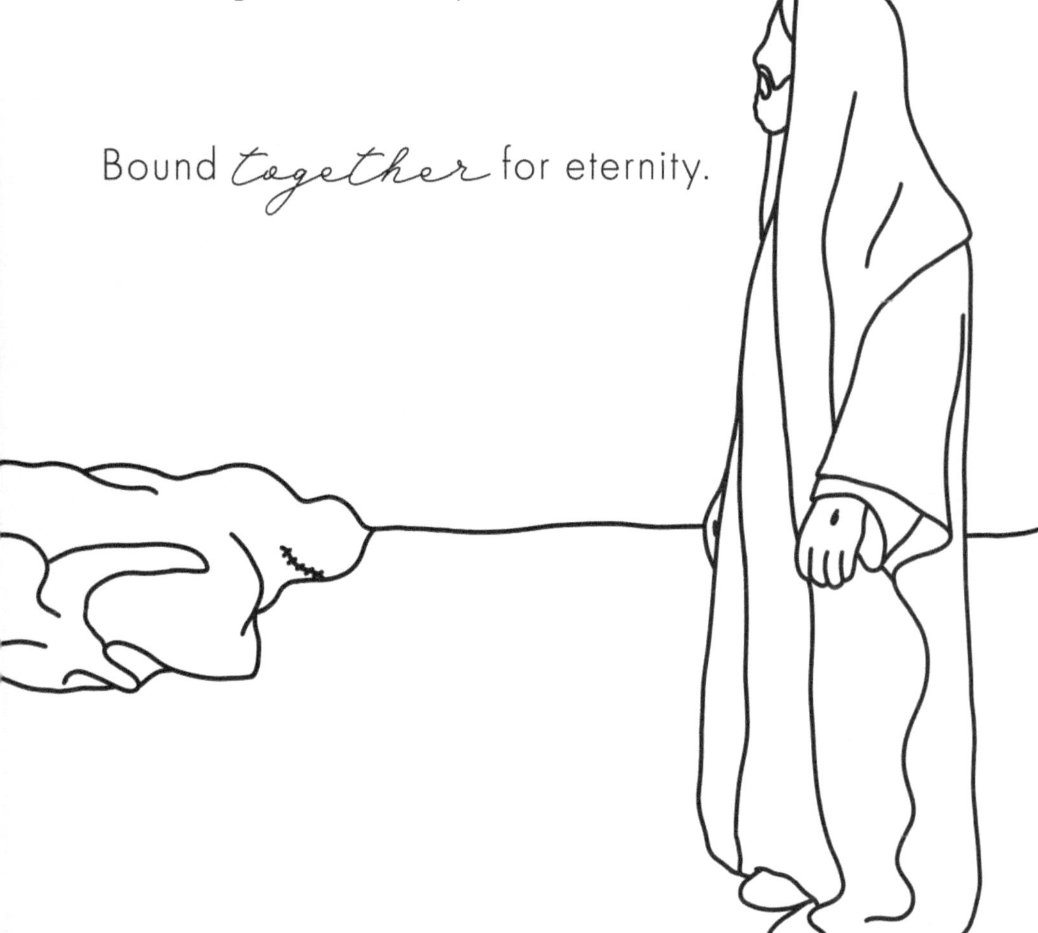

For now, I'll cuddle your *little ones,*
While they watch you from above.

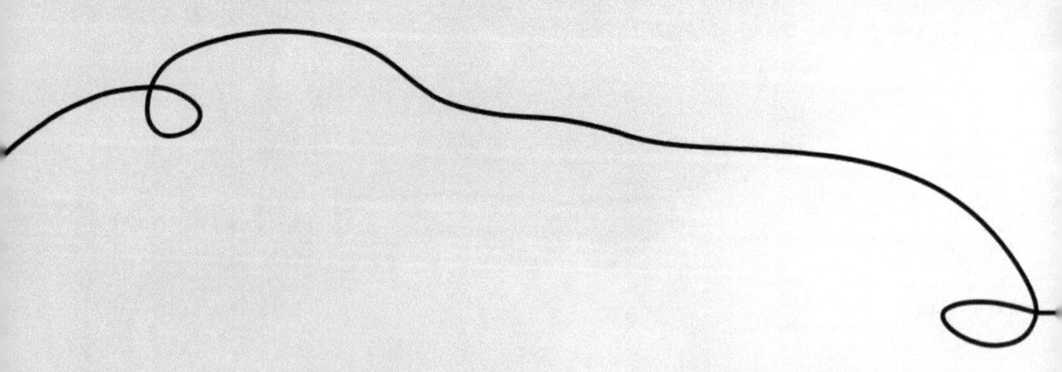

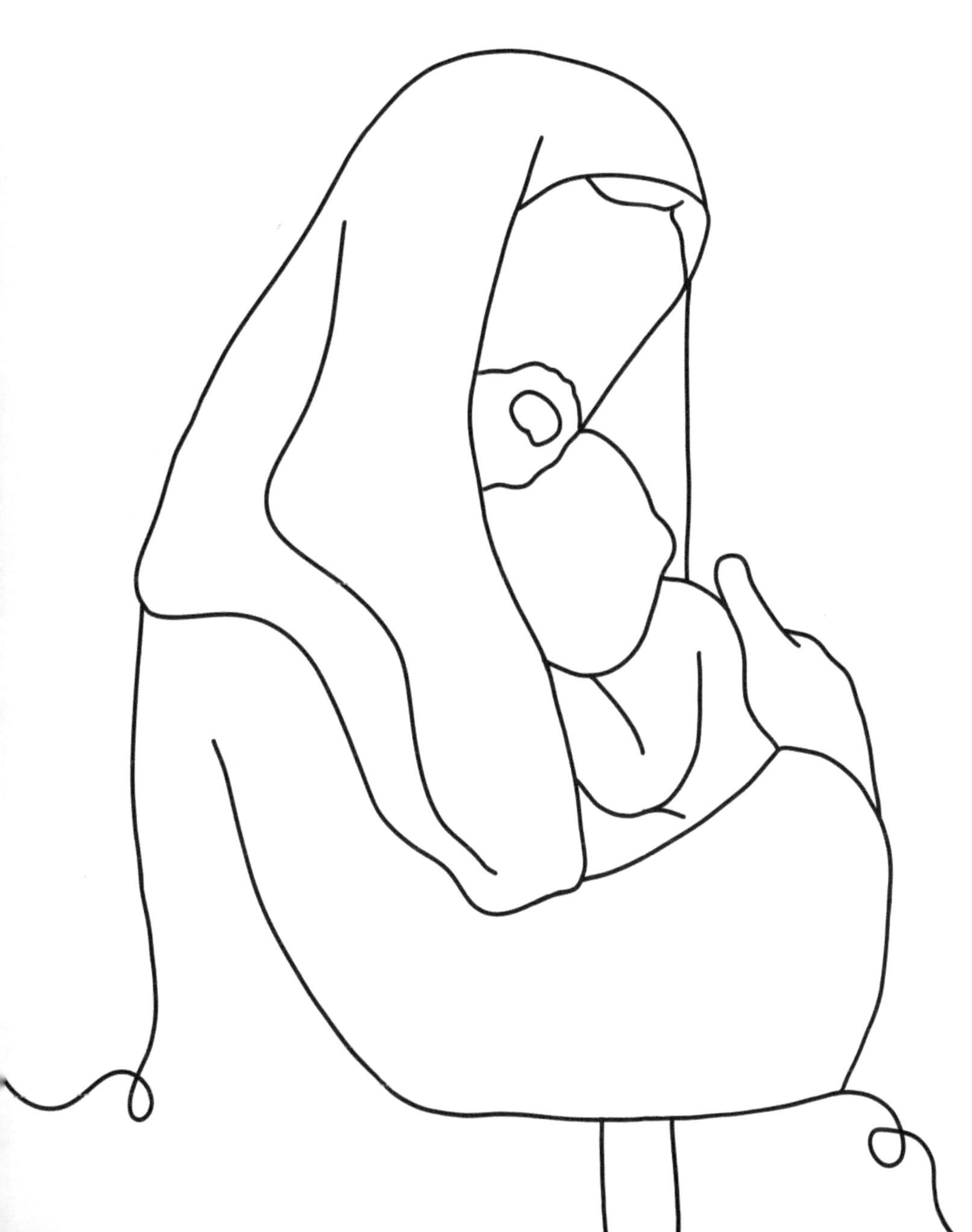

You will raise your babes one day,

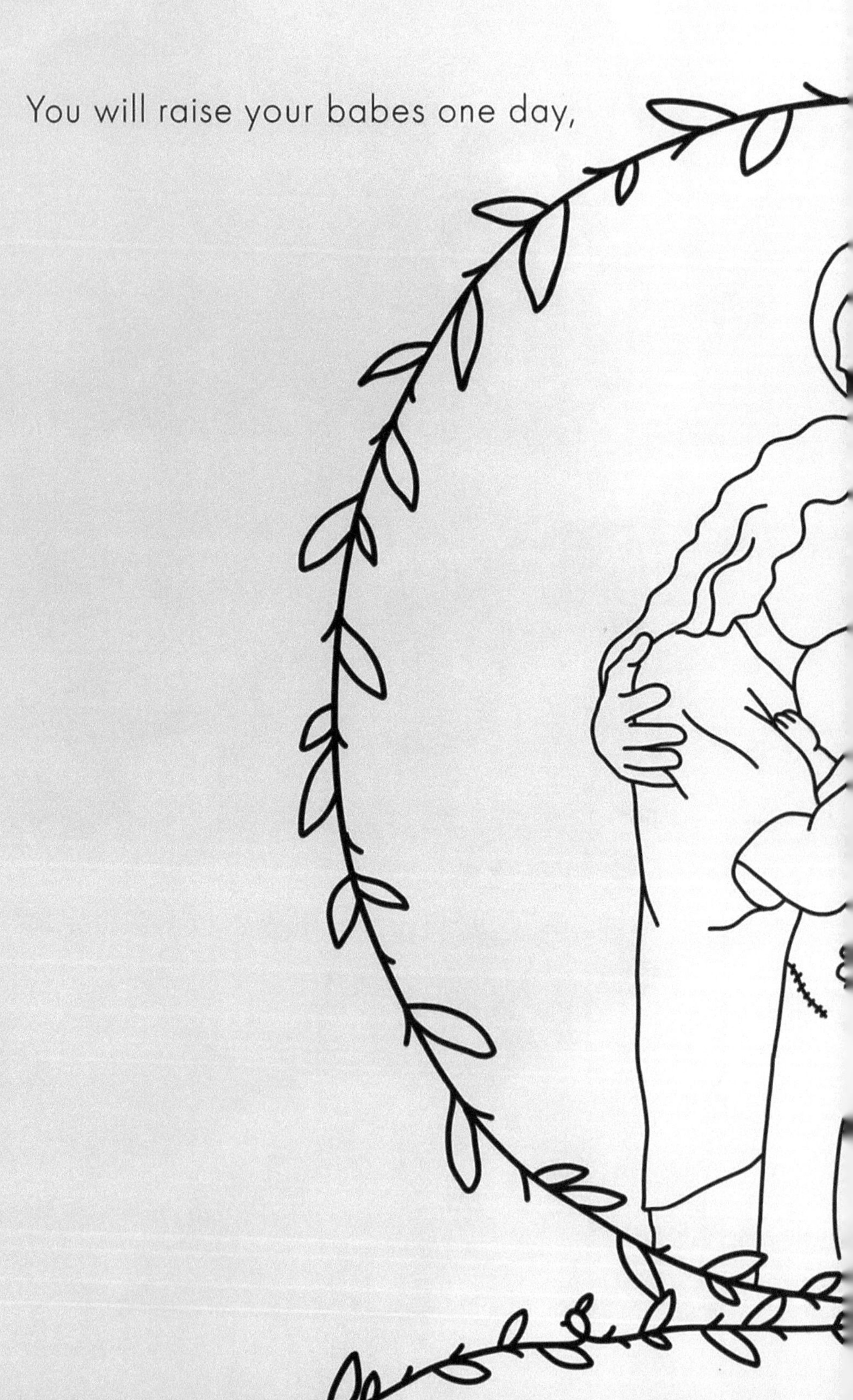

In a place of

beauty,

joy

and love.

thank you

I am forever grateful to my mother-in-law, Christine Thackeray. She lent an understanding ear to my tears and sought to help us however she could. Her writing experience gives this poem a true voice. The greatest word of wisdom she taught me during these years was this: It's okay to grieve, to be in and experience the darkness, but don't stay there. The longer you stay there, the harder it will be to climb out. Seek light in your life, even amidst your grief.

Thank you to my own mother, Marilyn Cottam. While she has never dealt with child loss, she has had her fair share of trials. Her ever-present love and never-ending hugs have given me comfort many a time over. And thank you to my two neighbors, my friends; who watched my children, bought me food, and gave me understanding shoulders to cry on. They were my village.

Thank you to my precious daughters. They have been my light during my darkest hours. They have given me a reason to seek light, to get up and not stay down, to press forward despite the blessings I lacked. They have been my constant reminder to cherish what I have and live in this moment.

And finally, thank you to my dear husband. You have had to carry more than you ever should. You have been my rock. You have helped me course correct and persevere. You have taught me deeper love and patience. You have helped me more than you know... as you continue to stand with me, without ceasing, even when we both feel weak, and support us through it all. I love you.

- Rachel Thackeray